THINK SAFETY – FIRST
Labels & Directions

THINK SAFETY -- FIRST	
Keep out of reach of children	
PRECAUTIONS Before opening this container	
Ventilation Needed	External Use Only
Wear eye protection	Wear protective clothing
CAUTION -- WARNING	
Harmful if swallowed	May cause breathing problems
Ingesting can be fatal	Eye and skin irritant
DANGER -- IN CASE OF ACCIDENT	
Call physician immediately	Fresh air is needed
Rinse eye with cool water	Rinse skin with running water
SAFE STORAGE	
Store in a cool, dry, locked cabinet or high shelf	
Combustible – Store away from flames and heat	
POISON CONTROL CENTER	

Jean Marie Miscisin, MLS, MA

I0436397

THINK SAFETY - FIRST
Labels & Directions

Copyright © 2012 Jean Marie Miscisin, MLS, MA

All Rights reserved to the Author.

ISBN: 10: 1477571396
ISBN: 13: 9781477571392

THINK SAFETY - FIRST
Labels & Directions

Cut health care cost by improving SAFETY LABELING on household products.

Reduce EMERGENCY ROOM VISITS by improving SAFETY LABELING.

With the cost of health care increasing REAL PREVENTIVE MESSURES can reduce the suffering from accidents and even deaths from improper use of toxic and volatile household products.

Currently there are Federal Laws regulating the information to be printed on the labels on products containing toxic poisonous chemicals.

There is a need for Standardized Safety LABELING with Consistent Formatting, Concise Statements, Easily Understood Wording, and Clear Directions.
Cover of this document is only one possible example.

The purpose of this book is to produce evidence that ALL ADULTS and the CHILDREN under their care are endangered when they do not read the labels of all household products before purchasing and using these products.

It is important in our American Society to read Labels and directions.

Most labels provide warnings, and directions. This information is important for living safely and for accident prevention. The lack of consistency in wording and placement of warnings on LABELS causes confusion at best to even good readers.

—

Adults with limited English proficiency are in even greater danger. They do not have access to these important avenues of information for living safely because:

They are not aware of the need to read labels and follow directions.
They do not realize that they do not understand the printed words and the importance to safe living. They do not know how to find meaning in the printed words.

They do not have access to information necessary to make safe decisions.
Without being able to read and understand printed words, adults with limited English proficiency and the minors under their care are living in unnecessary danger.

POISON CONTROL CENTER DATA

The following important information can be found in the document which is available on the internet:

2009 Annual Report of the American Association
of Poison Control Centers' National Poison
Data System (NPDS): 27th Annual Report

AAPCC 2009 Annual Report of the NPDS 991
Caller Site and Exposure Site
As shown in Table 2, of the 2,479,355 human exposures reported, 75.8% of the calls originated from a residence (own or other) but 93% actually occurred at a residence (own or other).

AAPCC 2009 Annual Report of the NPDS 993
Reason for Exposure
The reason for most human exposures was unintentional 2,043,155 (82.4%); unintentional general reason code was reported in 1,462,351 (59%) of all exposures (Table 6A).

These statistics alone should be enough evidence that there is a great need for Standardized Safety LABELING with Consistent Formatting, Concise Statements, Easily Understood Wording, and Clear Directions.

1. There is a great NEED for CONSISTENT and STANDARDIZED SAFETY LABELS on CLEANING and other PRODUCTS USED AROUND the HOME.

2. Yes, there are FEDERAL LAWS and FEDERAL STANDARDS for labeling dangerous products, if a person can find them and then adheres to the laws.

3. All of the PRECAUTIONS MUST BE PRINTED BEFORE the DIRECTIONS.

4. All of the WARNING, DANGER, and CAUTION INFORMATION should be printed following the PRECAUTIONS.

5. What should the person do IN CASE OF ACCIDENTS should be stated clearly.

6. STORAGE AND DISPOSAL INFORMATION should be indicated.

7. ALL of the DIRECTIONS have to be clearly IDENTIFIED, easily followed by the end user, and LOCATED in ONE PLACE on the LABEL.

I chose to use "real labels" from containers in order to provide accurate concrete evidence. These are products that I use from mostly brand name products.

The companies that recognize their products should take a good look at the labels on their products and make the changes voluntarily for the safety of the people who purchase and use their products.

What can we do?

READ ALL LABELS ON HOME CLEANING PRODUCTS is only the first step.

Before the labels are improved, all people can do their part by using this manual as a guide to reading labels and directions, so they can help themselves and their friends live more safely.

Write to your Senators and Congressman asking them, "When will they pass a law that requires consistent, standardized, SAFETY LABELING on household products?"
If possible, send a copy of this book, Think Safety – First.

Create an awareness of the need for better SAFETY LABELING LAWS by sending this book, Think Safety – First, to your friends and neighbors.

HOW TO USE THIS BOOK

Originally the purpose of this book was to integrate reading, writing, and communicating skills with analyzing, processing, and decision-making skills.

During the field research on the information in this book, participants found the following steps most helpful in learning how to live safely.

1. LOOK = What do I look for? Where should I look? What words are most important for safe living?

2. READ = What should I read? How should I read it?

3. MAKE MEANING (analyze) = Which words are KEY WORDS to help me understand this? Which words must go together to find the "real" meaning?

4. THINK (process) = What is this word telling me? What is this phrase telling me? What is this sentence telling me? What do I already know about these words?

5. DECIDE (action) = What is the safe thing to do? What would be a safe action when I see these words on a label? What would be the safest thing to do? What is the safest thing to do - when I don't understand what I read?

Real containers should be used for practice. Choose products that are available on local store shelves that are used for cleaning and taking care of the furniture, fixtures, and appliances in the home. I asked the participants to bring to class the cleaning products that they use in their homes. I also asked them to bring in containers with KEEP OUT OF REACH OF CHILDREN on the labels. Most of them brought in empty containers of various household products.

The participants in the field research were amazed at the lack of consistency in wording and placement of warnings on labels. These participants even suggested that we do a survey of product labels, and <u>start a petition to standardize warning labels on household cleaning products.</u>

This Book, Think Safety – First, is a start in the campaign for CONSISTENT and STANDARDIZED SAFETY LABELS on CLEANING PRODUCTS and other PRODUCTS USED AROUND the HOME.

GENERAL PRODUCT SAFETY LABEL
SAMPLE

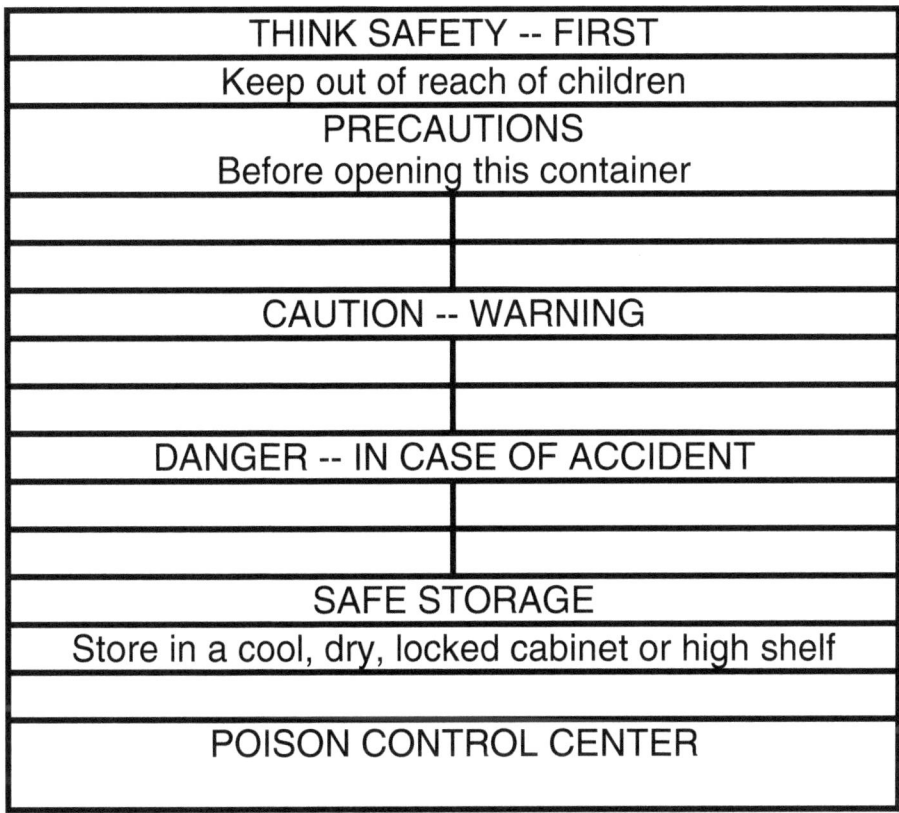

THINK SAFETY -- FIRST	
Keep out of reach of children	
PRECAUTIONS	
Before opening this container	
CAUTION -- WARNING	
DANGER -- IN CASE OF ACCIDENT	
SAFE STORAGE	
Store in a cool, dry, locked cabinet or high shelf	
POISON CONTROL CENTER	

Every company would then complete the information required for the SAFETY LABEL for each product that is sold in the United States of America.

This SAFETY LABEL would then be placed on the container label. This part of the label would be the first thing that the customer would read before purchasing the product. Then before opening the container the consumer would read the entire label and the more detailed DIRECTIONS.

—

READING AND INTERPRETING
CURRENT LABELS

Objectives:

- o   to introduce the vocabulary necessary for interpreting current labels,

- o   to create an awareness of meanings of phrases,
      Dictionary definitions only touch the surface of the implied meaning of many safety phrases.

- o   to practice applying actions or reactions to related words such as ventilate, ventilation, and ventilated.

- o   to elicit appropriate responses and behavior upon reading warnings on labels

- o   All of the LABEL words in this book came from actual labels on products brought to my classroom by adults who participated in the field research.

TOPICS

A. KEEP OUT OF REACH OF CHILDREN

B. WARNING, DANGER, CAUTION

C. DO NOT EAT! DO NOT DRINK!

D. FRESH AIR IS NEEDED!

E. PRECAUTIONS, PHRASES, AND OTHER WORDS

F. WRITTEN DIRECTIONS

What is a container?

Containers = Bottles, jars, cans, boxes, tubes, anything that hold a product used in and around the house and garage.

Where do you find the words: Warning, Caution, Precautions, Danger, etc.?

Where should a person look for information before opening a container?

Bottles = Read the label around the whole bottle. One spray bottle of window cleaner had directions and warnings on the back of the label that was stuck to the bottle so that a person had to "read through the liquid" to know how to use the product safely – making it nearly impossible for the best of readers.

Jars = Read the label on the jar. Read all printing on the lid and around the rim of the lid. Read the printing inside of the lid and any covering sealing the product.

Cans = Read the whole label. Turn the can on the side; sometimes there are Warnings printed sideways on the can.

Boxes = A person must look at the labels on all six (6) sides of a box … front, back, top, bottom, left side, and right side. Open the box and read the printing on the inside of the box. Read the sheet of paper with information that is usually enclosed.

Tubes = Most tubes come enclosed in boxes. Read all of the Directions, Precautions, and Warnings on the box. Read the sheet of paper with information that is usually enclosed in the box. Read the label on the tube. There could be precautions on the box, directions and possible side-affects on the sheet of paper, and additional directions and warnings on the tube.

TOPIC - A = Keep Out of Reach of Children
Cleaning products, medicines, pesticides, cosmetics

1. Look for the words, **Keep Out of Reach of Children**, on every **container** that holds products used in and around the house and garage.

2. When you see these words printed on a label, **Keep out of Reach of Children**, it means that the **contents could be dangerous**.

3. Read ALL LABELS, reading all the warnings and directions BEFORE OPENING the container.

4. When you **recognize** that these words are a **warning**, you know that something inside the container could hurt children, or you, if the contents are used for the wrong thing or in the wrong way.

5. Children are active, curious, and always getting into things.

6. Children are curious, like to explore, and try new things.

7. Special precautions must be taken when there are small children around.

8. Children should be taught to put only food in their mouths.

9. Do not store food items near containers that are labeled KEEP OUT OF REACH OF CHILDREN.

10. **Cleaning products** have this warning on the **labels**.

11. Cleaning products are always dangerous for small children.

12. Children like to shake things and chemicals can get in their eyes.

13. Children like to taste things and they can get very sick from just a taste of most cleaning products.

14. Products such as wax or paste for polishing furniture are also dangerous.

15. Cleaning products, pesticides, and polishing products in spray cans or aerosol cans can pose big problems for children and adults.

16. Children could breathe in toxic fumes or spray the contents in their eyes or noses.

17. For cockroaches and rodents, mice, rates, and gophers, there are pest killers that are in small pieces called pellets, and children can be POISONED by putting these pieces in their mouths.

18. **Garden chemicals** have this warning on the labels.

19. Liquid sprays used as fertilizer or for killing garden pests and bugs should also be kept out of reach of children.

20. Some garden liquids can hurt children's delicate and tender skin.

21. Automotive products had this warning on the labels.

22. Even hair coloring products have this warning on the labels.

23. Cosmetics may seem harmless, but children and adults may have severe skin reactions to them.

24. Powders can be harmful to children's and adults lungs.

25. Medicines have this warning on the labels.

26. MEDICINES can help a person get better, but too much medicine can kill a child.

27. The amount of medicine that can kill a child is much smaller than that which can kill an adult.

28. Measure medicine carefully – not too much, not too little.

29. Always follow the doctor's directions. If the directions are not clear ask the doctor to explain the directions using different words.

30. Nutritional supplements have this warning on the labels.

31. Products in containers with this label, **Keep Out of Reach of Children**, may have caps or lids that are difficult to open or special directions for opening them.

32. If you don't know how to use a product that had the label, **Keep out of Reach of Children**, ask a trusted friend to explain the words on the label or just don't purchase the product.

33. After using a product that is labeled with the warning, **Keep out of Reach of Children**, close the container carefully and promptly put the container in a safe place.

34. When possible, store containers with the warning, **Keep out of Reach of Children**, in locked cabinets, cupboards, or study chests.

35. The containers with the warning, **Keep out of Reach of Children**, should be stored on a high shelf, if they pose any danger to a child.

36. **Keep Out of Reach of Children**.

These are the most common dangers around the home and garage. Many new products that pose new dangers to consumers are coming to the stores every day.

TOPIC - B = WARNING, DANGER, CAUTION

1. Before opening a container, first look for the words, Keep Out of Reach of Children.

2. Before opening a box, look on all six sides for the words: **Warning, Danger**, and **Caution**.

3. The words, Warning, Danger, and Caution, all mean the same thing; something in the container can HURT you and your children.

4. WARNINGS may be printed on the **TOP, BOTTOM, FRONT, BACK, AND SIDES** of a box.

5. Look carefully on the labels of bottles, because the print may be small or even **SIDEWAYS**.

6. The words, **Warning, Danger**, and **Caution**, may be printed in a different color from the other printing on a label. RED is the most popular color.

7. The words, **Caution, Warning, and Danger**, may be printed in **BOLD DARK PRINT.**

8. OCCASIONALLY the words, **Danger, Caution, and Warning** are printed within the **DIRECTIONS** FOR USE.

9. Remember to read ALL the words in the sections of the label that have the titles: **Danger, Warning, and Caution.**

10. If you do not understand any of the words under the titles: **Warning, Danger**, and **Caution** on the label **DO NOT OPEN THE CONTAINER**.

11. Ask someone you trust to EXPLAIN the meaning of the words in the sections labeled: **Warning, Danger**, and **Caution**.

TOPIC - C = DO NOT EAT! DO NOT DRINK!

ALL of the following sentences mean that you should not eat, you should not drink, and you should not put the contents in your mouth. Do not let any of the contents get on food.

1. Do not take **internally**.

2. For **external** use only.

3. **Harmful** if swallowed.

4. **Avoid contact** with mucous membranes.

5. Do not **swallow**.

6. Avoid contact with food.

7. If accidentally swallowed **induce vomiting**.

8. If accidentally swallowed **do not induce vomiting**.

9. If accidentally **ingested call** a **physician** immediately.

10. If accidentally ingested drink mild and do not induce vomiting.

11. Ingesting this product can be harmful or **fatal**.

TOPIC - D = FRESH AIR IS NEEDED!

ALL of the following sentences mean use the product outside, open a window, open a door to outside air, and turn on a fan to blow fumes out of the house.
Before opening the container you may do one or more of these actions to provide FRESH OUTSIDE AIR.

1. Use in well ventilated area.

2. Provide adequate ventilation.

3. Do not use in closed area.

4. Avoid breathing vapors.

5. Avoid prolonged use.

6. Avoid inhalation.

7. Do not spray for longer than 90 seconds in one room.

8. Use outside.

9. Use out of doors.

10. Avoid inhalation of vapors.

11. Wear respiratory protection while using this product.

12. Open door or windows or use other mean to ensure fresh air entry during application and drying.

13. Toxic fumes.

14. Inhalation of this product has been shown to cause nerve and brain damage and in some instances have proven fatal.

15. Remove all food, plants, and pets before using this product.

16. After spraying this product do not reenter the room until the residue has settled out of the air.

TOPIC - E = PRECAUTIONS, PHRASES, AND OTHER WORDS

1. READ THE WHOLE LABEL BEFORE OPENING THE CONTAINER.

2. PRECAUTIONS may be listed in the DIRECTIONS.

3. Warnings may be printed within the directions. Example: Use only as directed.

4. Read all the directions before opening the container. Use only as directed.

5. Wear eye protection when using this product. Wear glasses or goggles when using the chemicals or sprays.

6. Fresh air is needed. Before opening the container … open a window. Open a door. Turn on a fan. Use out of doors. Use outside.

7. Respiratory protection is needed. Wear a gas mask, or air filtering mask.

8. Wear protective clothing. Wear a rubber apron or other clothing that is waterproof. Wear a mechanics coverall.

9. May cause skin irritation. Avoid contact with skin. Wear rubber or plastic gloves.

10. Do not incinerate. Do not put into fire.

11. Store away from heat. Put in a cool dry place. Keep away from heat.

12. Contents under pressure. The can could explode. Do not crush the container.

13. Flammable. Combustible. The contents could catch on fire easily.

14. Do not puncture. Do not punch a hole in the container.

15. Do not put into trash compactor.

16. Do not store above 120º (degrees Fahrenheit).

17. Store out of sun's rays.

18. Do not use on edible crops. Do not put the chemical on plants that are planted to produce food.

19. Avoid contamination of foodstuffs. Remove food from the room before opening the container. Cover food and place in a cupboard or other place that can be closed off from the sprays and chemicals.

TOPIC - F = WRITTEN DIRECTIONS

Objectives:

- o   to develop processing skills for understanding directions;

- o   to create an awareness of the importance of following directions;

- o   and to help define the dangers from not following directions carefully.

1.   When using cleaning products do not mix two products together.

2.   Try each one separately making sure that none of the first product remains on the toilet, floor, sink, or tile before trying another different product on the same place.

3.   When AMMONIA based products are mixed with products containing a CHEMICAL with the letters CHLOR, a POISONOUS GAS is formed that can kill a person.

4.   Look for the words DO NOT USE WITH AMMONIA on the label.

5.   Look on the label for the words DO NOT MIX WITH OTHER CLEANING PRODUCTS.

6.   Look for the words. Do not combine with AMMONIA based products.

7.   CHLOROX, CHLORIDE, CHLORINE, HYPOCHLORITE, and any word with the letters CHLOR should be a warning that the contents should be used carefully.

8.   DO NOT MIX CHLOR ... with any product that has AMMONIA or AMMONIUM written in the list of INGREDIENTS.

9. DO NOT MIX AMMONIA with any product that has the letters CHLOR in one of the INGREDIENTS.

10. FEDERAL LAW PROHIBITS USE OTHER THAN AS DIRECTED BY THE MANUFACTURER. Read all of the directions and follow them exactly.

11. Check the INGREDIENTS, the WARNINGS, and FOLLOW THE MANUFACTURER'S DIRECTIONS when using cleaning products.

12. Read the labels on containers of all products before you buy them.

13. Read all the warnings before you open the container and take the necessary precautions for your own safety.

14. Read all the directions before you use the product.

15. Follow all of the directions carefully.

A Librarian's wife developed brain cancer and died. Doctors suspected that Hair Coloring had caused the cancer so the Librarian opened a law suit against the manufacturer. The company even acknowledged that the hair coloring may have caused brain cancer. The company was not held liable because the woman had used the product more frequently than stated in the directions.

CRITERIA FOR JUDGING SAFETY OF LABELS

Three basic criteria were chosen for judging the sample labels included in this book.

1. Warnings and Directions are clearly identified.

2. The wording is concise and understood without difficulty.

3. Information can be easily located.

This book is requesting safer labeling and standardization to prevent accidents, personal injuries, poisonings, and fatalities from misunderstanding the information needed for proper use of products used in and around the home by the end consumer.

THREE CATEGORIES

GOOD LABELS:
These labels fulfill the requirements of all three criteria. The only factor missing is STANDARD LOCATION.

OKAY LABELS:
These labels fulfill the requirement of two of the criteria.

POOR LABELS:
These labels fulfill the requirements of one or none of the criteria.

LABELS – Where did you find these words?

Look at the labels on cleaning products and other liquids, sprays, powders, cosmetics, and other consumable products found in your home and your friends' homes.

Study the first SAMPLE CHART and then take your own product containers and fill in the second chart.

All dangerous products are required by law to have warnings on the LABELS ... YOU have to look carefully before you buy them.

LOOK = Where should I look? = SAMPLE CHART

Products	Keep Out of Reach of Children	Warning	Danger	Caution
Bleach Big Bottle	Front of bottle	Small hard to read = three places on label	Big words = Two places	Not on this label.
Bug Spray Can	Front	Back = small print		Front and back of can in with the Directions
Oven Cleaner	Back			Front and back
Powdered Cleaner	Down the side>	very hard to >	read.	Front

LOOK = Where should I look?

Products	Keep Out of Reach of Children	Warning	Danger	Caution

LABELS - SAFE THING TO DO

Read the labels before opening the container.
What is a safe preventive action?
If possible read the LABELS before purchasing all products.
Choose the safest products to protect your family and YOU.
All dangerous products are required by law to have warnings on the
LABEL-- YOU have to look carefully before you buy them.
If you need help ask a trusted friend to explain the labeling.

Words on the LABEL	Safe Thing to DO
… induce vomiting …	
… do not induce vomiting …	
… fatal …	
… ventilation …	
… toxic fumes …	
… ingested …	
… call physician …	
… combustible …	
… inhalation …	
… nerve damage …	
… avoid contact …	
… inflammable/ flammable …	
… brain injury …	
… external use …	
… harmful vapors …	
… skin irritation …	

GOOD LABEL
RELIEVES PAIN AND ITCH

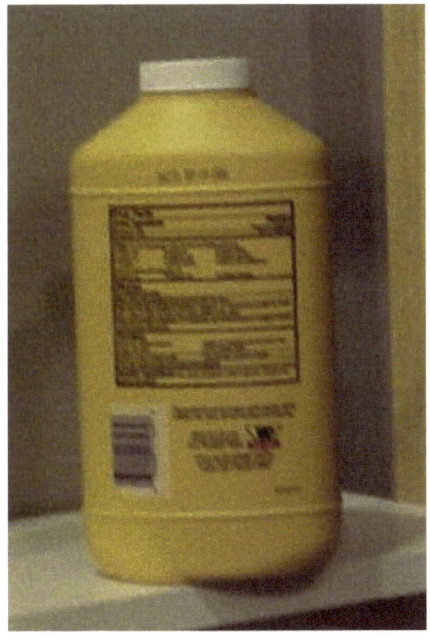

1. Information can be easily located. YES!
    Information in one place and placed in a table format.

2. Warnings and Directions are clearly identified. YES!
    Warnings: are located before the Directions.

3. The wording is concise and understood without difficulty.
    YES!   Each warning is in a separate section on the table.

Warnings:
For external use only
When using this product avoid contact with eyes
Stop use and ask a doctor if condition worsens, or if symptoms persist for more than 7 days or clear up and occur again within a few days
Keep out of reach of children. If swallowed get medical help or contact a Poison Control Center right away

―

GOOD LABEL
Hydrogen Peroxide

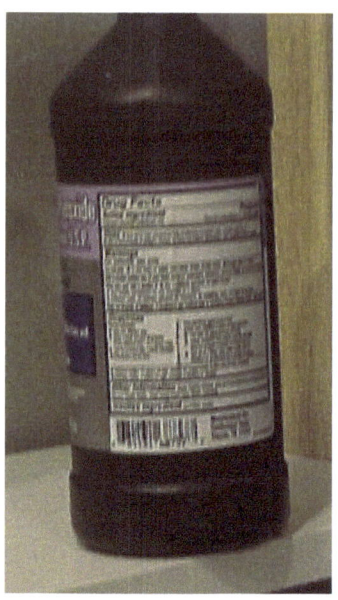

1. Information can be easily located. YES!
    Information in one place and placed in a table format.
2. Warnings and Directions are clearly identified. YES!
    Warnings: are located before the Directions.
3. The wording is concise and understood without difficulty.
    YES!   Each warning is in a separate section on the table.

Warnings: **For external use only**
Do not use • in the eyes or over large areas of the body • longer than one week
Ask a doctor before use if you have deep or puncture wounds, animal bites or serious burns
Stop use and ask a doctor if • the condition persists or gets worse • sore mouth symptoms do not improve in 7 days (use as a rinse only) • irritation, pain or redness persists or worsens • swelling, rash, or fever develops
Keep out of reach of children.   If swallowed get medical help or contact a Poison Control Center right away.

GOOD LABEL
Leather Lotion

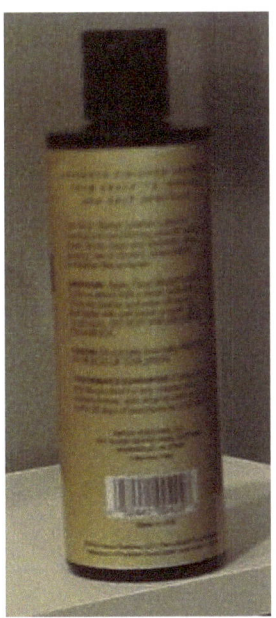

1. Information can be easily located. YES!
   All information is on back label.

2. Warnings and Directions are clearly identified. YES!
   The word CAUTION is clearly indicated and is printed below
   the DIRECTIONS.

3. The wording is concise and understood without difficulty.
   YES!   CAUTION: Do not take Internally.

KEEP OUT OF REACH OF CHILDREN.

OKAY LABEL
General Household Cleaner

On the front label one can find in clear, yellow lettering "Non-Toxic."

On the very bottom of the front label in thin, white lettering are these words:
"CAUTION: MILD EYE IRRITANT – See back panel for additional precautionary statements."
I kept the proportions as near to the label, however all of them are slightly smaller than are presented here.

Back Label

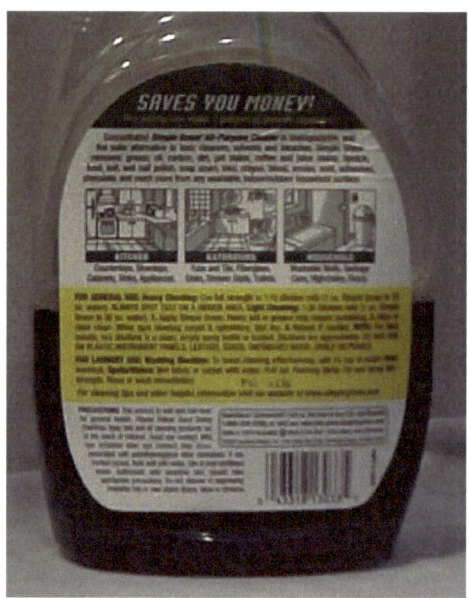

1. Information can be easily located. OKAY!
   All of the PRECAUTIONS are in one place on the label.
   They are in very small print.

2. Warnings and Directions are clearly identified. OKAY!
   "PRECAUTIONS" on the left at the bottom of the label.

The next page will provide more details.

PRECAUTIONS

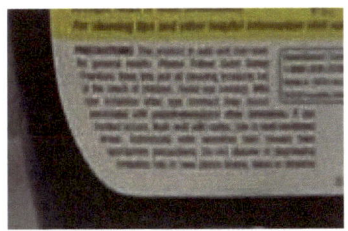

This picture is near actual size.

PRECAUTIONS: This product is safe and non-toxic for general health.

Please Follow Good Safety Practices. (These words are in italics.) Keep this and all cleaning products out of the reach of children. Avoid eye contact. Mild eye irritation after eye contact may occur associated with polyethyleneglycol ether derivatives. If eye contact occurs, flush well with water.

Use in well ventilated areas. Individuals with sensitive skin should take appropriate precautions. Do not dispose of degreasing rinseates into or near storm drains, lakes, or streams.

3. The wording is concise and understood without difficulty.
   NO!
   Many of the words are unfamiliar to most users of this product.
   The Precautions are at the bottom of the label instead of in a prominent location.

OKAY LABEL
Detergent for Hand Washing Dishes

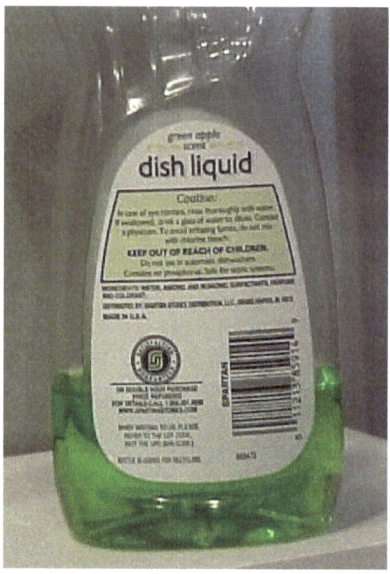

1. Information can be easily located. YES!
   All information is on back label.

2. Warnings and Directions are clearly identified.
   The word caution clearly indicated. YES!
   One warning states,
"To avoid irritating fumes, do not mix with chlorine bleach."
   OKAY!

3. The wording is concise and understood without difficulty.
   NO!   There are no specific directions on
          "how to use" this product.
   The statement, "Do not use in automatic dishwashers,"
          is on the bottom of the Caution label.

OKAY LABEL
Wax for Cleaning and Caring for Wood

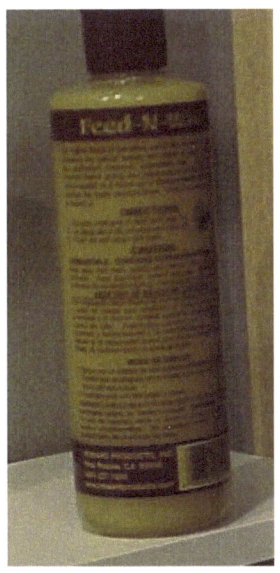

1. Information can be easily located. YES!
   CAUTION: COMBUSTIBLE –
   Read other cautions on back panel.

2. Warnings and Directions are clearly identified. YES!
   On the back panel the word CAUTION is clearly indicated.
   DIRECTIONS are printed above CAUTION.

3. The wording is concise and understood without difficulty.
   NO!   Some difficult words under CAUTION =
   COMBUSTIBLE: CONTAINS PETROLEUM DISTILLATE.
   In small print = Keep away from heat, sparks, and flame.
   Use with adequate ventilation.
   Avoid prolonged contact with skin.
   FIRST AID: If swallowed, do not induce vomiting.
   Call physician immediately.
   KEEP OUT OF REACH OF CHILDREN –
    is printed and underlined.

OKAY LABEL
Furniture Polish

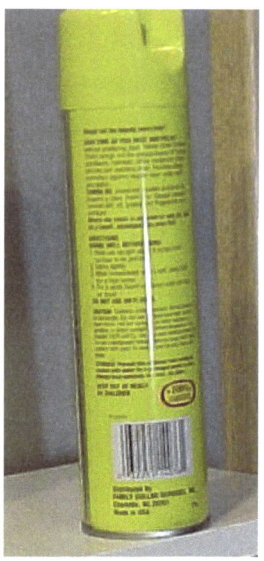

1. Information can be easily located. YES!
   CAUTION: CONTENTS UNDER PRESSURE –
   Read precautions on back of can.

2. Warnings and Directions are clearly identified. YES!
   On back of can the word CAUTION is clearly indicated.
   DIRECTIONS are printed above the word CAUTION.

3. The wording is concise and understood without difficulty.
   NO!   CAUTION is lengthy, detailed, and several warnings
   in one paragraph with run-on sentences.

"Contents under pressure. Do not puncture or incinerate.
Do not store near heat, sparks, open flame, red hot surfaces, or
other sources of ignition, in direct sunlight or where temperature will
exceed 120º F (49º C) Use in well ventilated area only.
Do not intentionally inhale vapor or spray mist.
Avoid contact with eyes. In case of eye contact, flush with water."

KEEP OUT OF REACH OF CHILDREN – is printed after
STORAGE just above the bar code at the bottom of the can.

OKAY LABEL
Laundry Detergent

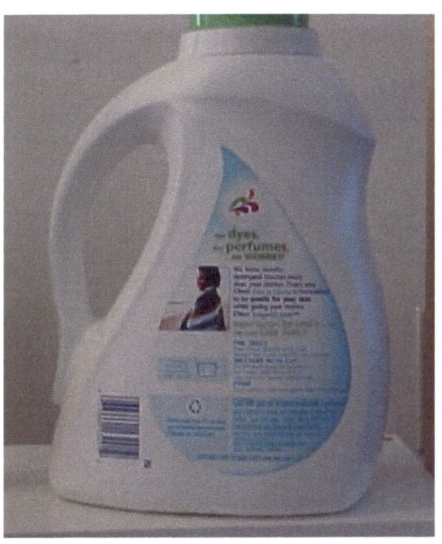

1. Information can be easily located. OKAY!
   Front label blue print on blue color section.
   CAUTION: EYE IRRITANT.
   HARMFUL IF SWALLOWED.
   SEE CAUTION ON BACK PANEL.

2. Warnings and Directions are clearly identified. OKAY!
   On the back panel the blue on blue print impedes clarity and
   reduces the importance of the message.

3. The wording is concise and understood without difficulty.
   OKAY!   CAUTION: KEEP OUT OF REACH OF CHILDREN.
   If swallowed, give a glass or water. Call a physician.
   In case of eye contact, flush with water.
   DO NOT REUSE THIS PACKAGE FOR DISPENSING
   BEVERAGES OR OTHER LIQUIDS.

POOR LABEL - BLEACH

FOLLOWING DIRECTIONS on LABELS including "chlor-words;"
Original Size is extremely difficult to read.

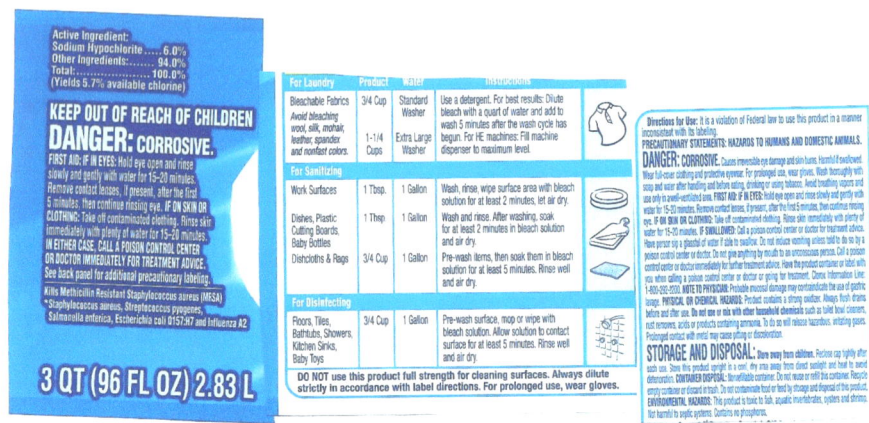

This label is very close to actual size of the label.
For the purposes of this book, the three parts are enlarged.
Each section is discussed in greater detail on the following pages.

1. Warnings and Directions are clearly identified. NO!
   Although there are "Warnings" on the label –

   ## They are not clearly identified.
   Directions are identified; however some of the "Warnings"
   are printed at the bottom of the section with directions.

2. The wording is concise and understood without difficulty.
   NO1
   KEEP OUT OF REACH OF CHILDREN begins one of the
   sections of warnings.
   Then gives information of what to do in case of accidents.

3. Information can be easily located. NO!
   Definitely not – the section labeled,
   "Directions for Use" states:
   "It is a violation of Federal law to use this product in a
   manner inconsistent with its labeling." Then instead of giving
   directions, the next line of this part of the label states:
   "PRECAUTIONARY STATEMENTS: HAZZARDS TO HUMANS
   AND DOMESTIC ANIMALS."

The above three parts to one label are enlarged so YOU can read ALL of the directions and the Dangers connected with using this BLEACH product.

PART 1

ACTIVE INGREDIENT: HYPOCHLORITE
IMPORTANT PART = CHLORITE

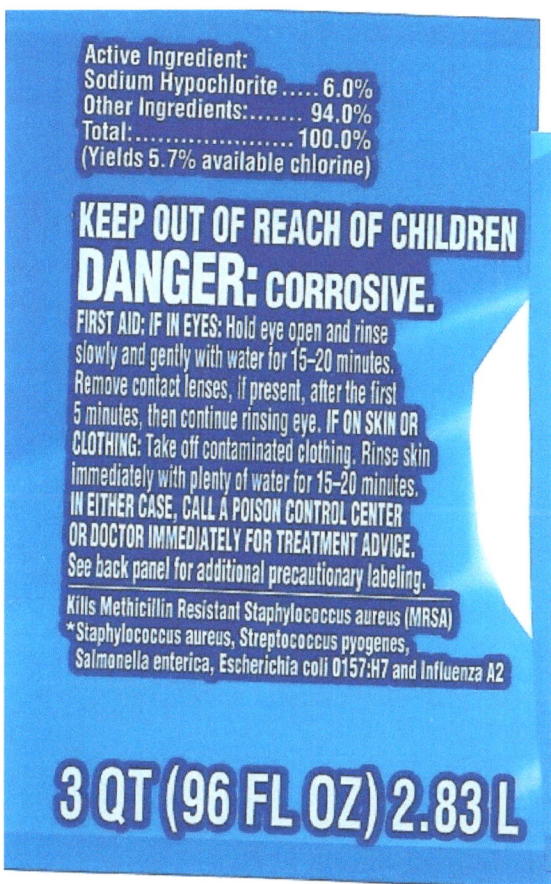

PART 2

DIRECTIONS FOR USE
SEE WARNING AT THE BOTTOM OF PART 2
SEE DANGERS ON PART 3

THIS ONE BLEACH PRODUCT CONTAINS MANY WARNINGS
ON DIFFERENT PARTS OF THE LABEL
THE SAFEST ACTION IS TO BUY A SAFER PRODUCT

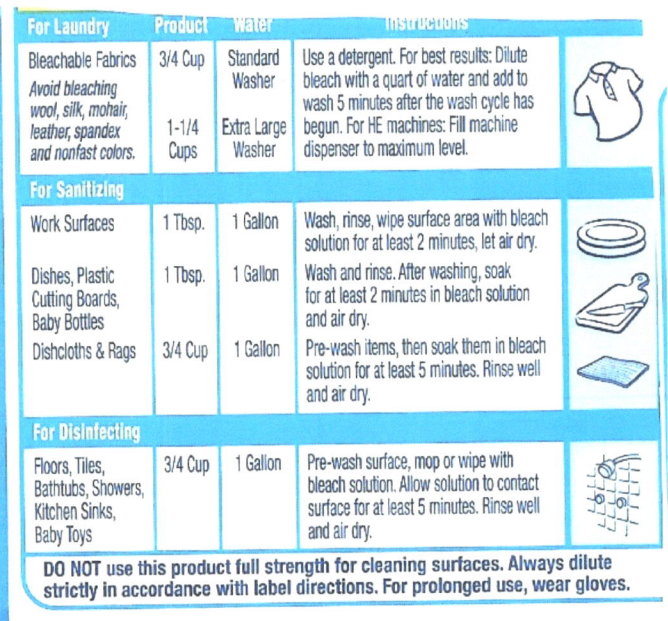

For Laundry	Product	Water	Instructions	
Bleachable Fabrics *Avoid bleaching wool, silk, mohair, leather, spandex and nonfast colors.*	3/4 Cup 1-1/4 Cups	Standard Washer Extra Large Washer	Use a detergent. For best results: Dilute bleach with a quart of water and add to wash 5 minutes after the wash cycle has begun. For HE machines: Fill machine dispenser to maximum level.	
For Sanitizing				
Work Surfaces	1 Tbsp.	1 Gallon	Wash, rinse, wipe surface area with bleach solution for at least 2 minutes, let air dry.	
Dishes, Plastic Cutting Boards, Baby Bottles	1 Tbsp.	1 Gallon	Wash and rinse. After washing, soak for at least 2 minutes in bleach solution and air dry.	
Dishcloths & Rags	3/4 Cup	1 Gallon	Pre-wash items, then soak them in bleach solution for at least 5 minutes. Rinse well and air dry.	
For Disinfecting				
Floors, Tiles, Bathtubs, Showers, Kitchen Sinks, Baby Toys	3/4 Cup	1 Gallon	Pre-wash surface, mop or wipe with bleach solution. Allow solution to contact surface for at least 5 minutes. Rinse well and air dry.	

DO NOT use this product full strength for cleaning surfaces. Always dilute strictly in accordance with label directions. For prolonged use, wear gloves.

This part of the label states, "Always dilute strictly in accordance with label directions."

SEE THE NEXT PART OF THE LABEL WHICH STATES:
"Directions for Use: it is a violation of Federal law to use this product in a manner inconsistent with its labeling."

NOTE AT THE BOTTOM OF NEXT LABEL UNDER "DANGER":
"Do not mix with other household chemicals such as toilet bowl cleaners, rust removers, acids or products containing ammonia. To do so will release hazardous, irritating gases."

VERY IMPORTANT INFORMATION
DANGER and PRECAUTIONARY STATEMENTS
STORAGE and DISPOSAL

Directions for Use: It is a violation of Federal law to use this product in a manner inconsistent with its labeling.
PRECAUTIONARY STATEMENTS: HAZARDS TO HUMANS AND DOMESTIC ANIMALS.

DANGER: CORROSIVE. Causes irreversible eye damage and skin burns. Harmful if swallowed. Wear full-cover clothing and protective eyewear. For prolonged use, wear gloves. Wash thoroughly with soap and water after handling and before eating, drinking or using tobacco. Avoid breathing vapors and use only in a well-ventilated area. **FIRST AID: IF IN EYES:** Hold eye open and rinse slowly and gently with water for 15–20 minutes. Remove contact lenses, if present, after the first 5 minutes, then continue rinsing eye. **IF ON SKIN OR CLOTHING:** Take off contaminated clothing. Rinse skin immediately with plenty of water for 15–20 minutes. **IF SWALLOWED:** Call a poison control center or doctor for treatment advice. Have person sip a glassful of water if able to swallow. Do not induce vomiting unless told to do so by a poison control center or doctor. Do not give anything by mouth to an unconscious person. Call a poison control center or doctor immediately for further treatment advice. Have the product container or label with you when calling a poison control center or doctor or going for treatment. Clorox Information Line: 1-800-292-2200. **NOTE TO PHYSICIAN:** Probable mucosal damage may contraindicate the use of gastric lavage. **PHYSICAL OR CHEMICAL HAZARDS:** Product contains a strong oxidizer. Always flush drains before and after use. **Do not use or mix with other household chemicals** such as toilet bowl cleaners, rust removers, acids or products containing ammonia. To do so will release hazardous, irritating gases. Prolonged contact with metal may cause pitting or discoloration.

STORAGE AND DISPOSAL: Store away from children. Reclose cap tightly after each use. Store this product upright in a cool, dry area away from direct sunlight and heat to avoid deterioration. **CONTAINER DISPOSAL:** Nonrefillable container. Do not reuse or refill this container. Recycle empty container or discard in trash. Do not contaminate food or feed by storage and disposal of this product. **ENVIRONMENTAL HAZARDS:** This product is toxic to fish, aquatic invertebrates, oysters and shrimp. Not harmful to septic systems. Contains no phosphorus.

1. Warnings and Directions are clearly identified. NO!
   Although the heading is clearly identified, there are many "DANGERS" and one is not distinguished from another.

2. The wording is concise and understood without difficulty. NO!
   The sentences contain large complicated wording.

3. Information can be easily located. NO!
   A person would have to read several sentences before reading =
"Do not mix with other household chemicals such as toilet bowl cleaners, rust removers, acids or products containing ammonia. To do so will release hazardous, irritating gases."

37

MANY IMPORTANT WORDS ARE ON THIS SMALL SECTION
PART 3 OF THE LABEL

First Line = Directions for Use: It is a violation of Federal law to use
      this product in a manner inconsistent with its labeling.

The "Directions" do not follow this First Line, as would be the logical
and responsible place to find them.

The "Directions" are found on different parts of the label and are
confusing at best.

Finally, a person could be in legal trouble by "violation of Federal
law" if that person gets hurt or worse yet by hurting of killing
somebody else by not following the "Directions" as printed on the
label.

This one product can cause harm to a person because the
"Directions" are confusing and easily misunderstood including a
person who reads English, and who understands most difficult
words by using a dictionary.

Second Statement = PRECAUTIONARY STATEMENTS:
      HAZARDS TO HUMANS AND DOMESTIC ANIMALS.

The person who understands these printed English words will then
read the difficult, and confusing words in the section under the
heading: DANGER: CORROSIVE.

The greatest DANGER can come if the consumer does not follow this direction =

"Do not mix with other household chemicals such as toilet bowl cleaners, rust removers, acids or products containing ammonia." The label only warns: "To do so will release hazardous, irritating gases."

Chlor-

One of the participants with limited English proficiency brought in the labels from this product and a product containing ammonia and related this frightening incident.

A person with limited experience with cleaning a toilet asked two neighbors what they used to clean their toilets.

One neighbor used an all-purpose cleaner with ammonia, so the individual tried to clean the toilet with that product.

Still the toilet was not very clean.

The other neighbor suggested bleach so the person went home and cleaned the toilet with bleach.

The toilet still didn't look clean.

So this adult, who couldn't understand the directions on the containers, in an effort to get the toilet really clean, sprayed the toilet with the all-purpose cleaner with ammonia and then poured in some bleach. Inside the toilet the liquids started to make a sizzling noise and suddenly the toilet exploded.

The person took the hand of the small child who also lived in the house and they both ran outside. This action prevented the child from getting hurt. The adult had a very bad headache, but was lucky to be alive.

—

1. What caused the explosion in the toilet?

2. What caused the adult to get a headache?

3. What precautions should a person take before using cleaning products?

4. What are some safe actions that could prevent accidents when cleaning toilets?

5. What are some general safe actions when using other household products for cleaning or maintenance?

What are some general safe actions when using chemicals in and around the house?

What are some general safe actions when using chemicals in and around the garage?

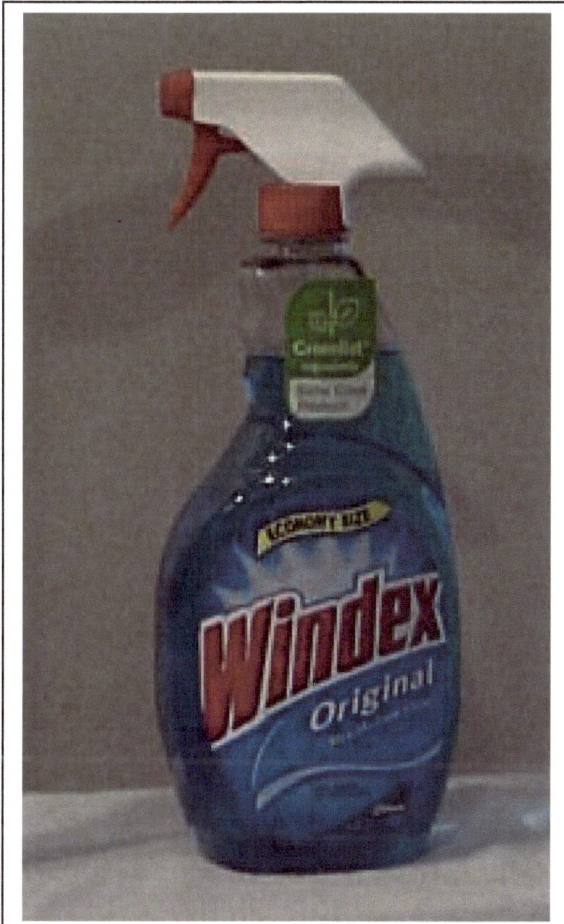

Front Label:
This product has the words in fine print at the very bottom of the bottle underneath the light blue wave: "Glass cleaner with Ammonia D" and no further warning.

See the next picture.

This company expects the customer to read through the "BLUE LIQUID" for directions and warnings if any.

The print is distorted by the liquid and so I gave up.

For most people who don't even try the danger increases.

<<<<< "Glass Cleaner with Ammonia D."

GLASS CLEANER

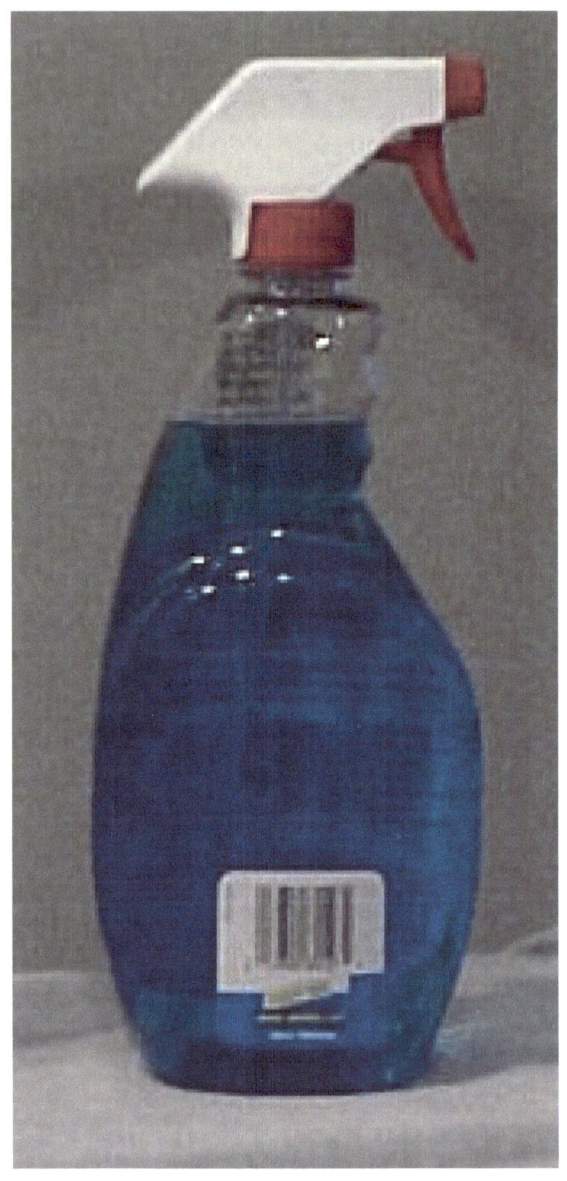

Back of Bottle

POOR LABEL
Spray Paint

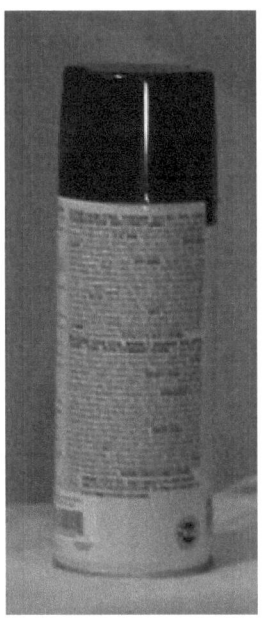

1. Information can be easily located. = NO!
   Front label ½ inch high 1 ½ inch long there are 5 (five) lines of very small print. Warnings overlap lines.
   This small font is twice the size of the print on the can.
   DANGER: EXTREMELY FLAMMABLE! VAPORS MAY CAUSE FLASH FIRES! CONTENTS UNDER PRESSURE. VAPOR HARMFUL. IRRITATES EYES, SKIN, AND RESPIRATORY TRACT.
   Before using carefully read CAUTIONS on back panel.

2. Warnings and Directions are clearly identified. NO!
   Twenty (20) lines of Warnings are compacted into a section of the label 2 inches high by 2 ½ inches long.
   The Directions are equally difficult to read.

3. The wording is concise and understood without difficulty. NO!   Back panel is extremely difficult to read because of small print and no separation between different DANGERS. The print below is much larger than the actual print.

... Keep area ventilated during use and until all vapors are gone. ... VAPOR HARMFUL. May affect the brain or nervous system causing dizziness, headache, or nausea. Causes eye, eye, skin, nose and throat irritation. Avoid continuous breathing of vapor and spray mist. ... NOTICE: Reports have associated repeated and prolonged occupational over exposure to solvents with permanent brain and nervous system brain damage. Intentional misuse by deliberately concentrating and inhaling the contents may be harmful or fatal.

On the bottom of the can next to the Bar Code:
WARNING: This product contains chemicals known to the State of California to cause cancer and birth defects or other reproductive harm.

POOR LABEL
CARB AND CHOKE CLEANER

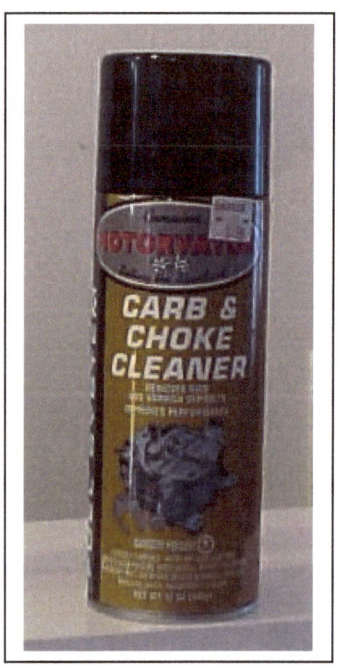

Front Label:
White print on gold can =
The following is compressed into two single inch long lines:
DANGER POISON! with the Skull and Cross-bones symbol.
EXTREMELY FLAMMABLE – VAPORS MAY CAUSE FLASH FIRES.
CONTENTS UNDER PRESSURE.
VAPOR HARMFUL. IRRITATES EYES, SKIN, AND RESPIRATORY TRACT.
MAY BE FATAL OR CAUSE BLINDNESS IF SWALLOWED.
Before using read CAUTIONS on back panel.

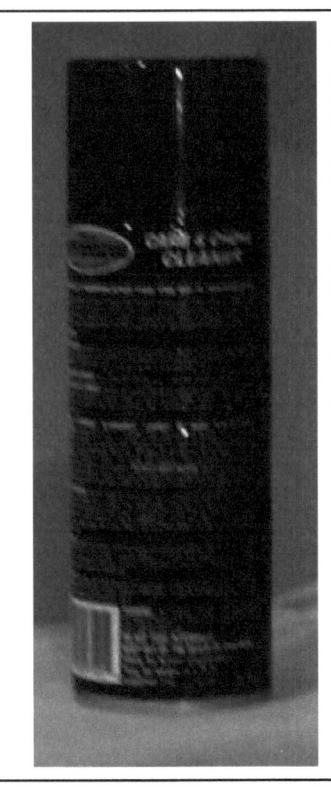

Back Panel:
Gray print on black can =
The following is compressed into two inch long lines:
This can is extremely dangerous. ...
NOTICE: Reports have associated repeated and prolonged occupational exposure to solvents with permanent brain and nervous system damage.

Back Panel Continued:
Intentional misuse by deliberately concentrating and inhaling the contents may be harmful or fatal.

The words above and below are in very small print. On the base of the can next to the Bar Code:

WARNING: This product contains chemicals known to the State of California to cause cancer and birth defects or other reproductive harm.

Now that YOU have this important information –
It is up to YOU.

SO ?????

WHAT ARE YOU GOING TO DO NEXT???

www.ingramcontent.com/pod-product-compliance
Lightning Source LLC
Chambersburg PA
CBHW040315010626
45792CB00022B/500